DR. BARBARA JUICING RECIPES FOR DIABETES

Discover Dr. Barbara's delicious juicing recipes for diabetes cure. Transform your health with nutrient-rich beverages for a healthier life

Miguel Sofia

Table of Contents

CHAPTER ONE 4

Introduction to Dr. Barbara's Holistic Approach to Managing Diabetes with Herbal Juicing 4

Understanding Diabetes 5

Conventional Management of Diabetes 5

The Role of Herbal Juicing in Diabetes Management 6

Herbs for Diabetes Management 6

Preparing Herbal Juices 8

Incorporating Herbal Juices into Daily Routine 8

Conclusion 9

CHAPTER TWO 10

Understanding Diabetes: Dr. Barbara's Insights into the Disease and Its Impact on Health 10

The Physiology of Diabetes 11

Impact on Health and Well-being 12

Dr. Barbara's Approach to Diabetes Management 13

CHAPTER THREE 16

The Healing Power of Herbal Juicing: How Fresh Juices Can Support Diabetes Control 16

Understanding Herbal Juicing 17

Herbs and Vegetables for Diabetes Control 17

- Mechanisms of Action 19
- Conclusion 22
- **CHAPTER FOUR** 22
  - Preparing for Your Juicing Journey: Setting Goals and Gathering Ingredients 22
  - Setting Clear Goals 23
  - Selecting Ingredients for Juicing 24
  - Preparing Your Juicing Station 25
  - Conclusion 26
- **CHAPTER FIVE** 27
  - Selecting the Right Herbs: Dr. Barbara's Recommended Ingredients for Juicing to Manage Diabetes 27
- **CHAPTER SIX** 31
  - Crafting Healing Recipes: Juices Designed to Stabilize Blood Sugar Levels and Promote Wellness 31
  - Conclusion 37
- **CHAPTER SEVEN** 38
  - Incorporating Additional Nutrients: Enhancing the Nutritional Value of Your Juices for Diabetes Management 38
  - Conclusion 41
- **CHAPTER EIGHT** 42

Navigating Challenges: Tips for Adjusting to Juicing and Managing Blood Sugar Fluctuations 42

Conclusion 46

CHAPTER NINE 47

Success Stories: Real-Life Accounts of Individuals Who Have Improved Their Diabetes Through Herbal Juicing 47

Conclusion 50

CHAPTER TEN 51

Beyond Juicing: Integrating Dr. Barbara's Principles for Long-Term Diabetes Management and Overall Health 51

Conclusion 54

THE END 83

COPYRIGHT © 2023

All rights reserved. No part of this publication may be reproduced, distributed, or transmitted in any form or by any means, including photocopying, recording, or other electronic or mechanical methods, without the prior written permission of the publisher, except in the case of brief quotations embodied in critical reviews and certain other noncommercial uses permitted by copyright law.

CHAPTER ONE

Introduction to Dr. Barbara's Holistic Approach to Managing Diabetes with Herbal Juicing

Dr. Barbara's holistic approach to managing diabetes with herbal juicing encompasses a comprehensive strategy that integrates various natural remedies, dietary adjustments, and lifestyle changes to support individuals in effectively managing their diabetes. In recent years, there has been a growing interest in alternative and complementary therapies for chronic conditions like diabetes, as people seek ways to enhance their well-being beyond conventional medical interventions. Dr. Barbara's approach emphasizes the use of herbal juicing as a key component of this holistic strategy, harnessing the therapeutic properties of herbs to promote blood sugar regulation, improve insulin sensitivity, and enhance overall health.

Understanding Diabetes

Before delving into Dr. Barbara's holistic approach, it's essential to understand the nature of diabetes and its impact on the body. Diabetes is a chronic metabolic disorder characterized by elevated levels of blood glucose (sugar) resulting from either inadequate insulin production, ineffective insulin action, or both. Insulin, produced by the pancreas, is a hormone that regulates blood sugar levels by facilitating the uptake of glucose into cells for energy production or storage. In individuals with diabetes, this regulatory mechanism is impaired, leading to persistent hyperglycemia (high blood sugar) which, if left uncontrolled, can contribute to various complications affecting the eyes, kidneys, nerves, and cardiovascular system.

Conventional Management of Diabetes

The conventional management of diabetes typically revolves around medication, dietary modifications, regular exercise, and monitoring of blood sugar levels. Medications may include oral hypoglycemic agents to lower blood sugar levels or insulin therapy for those with Type 1 diabetes or advanced Type 2 diabetes. Dietary recommendations often emphasize carbohydrate counting, portion control, and choosing foods with a low glycemic index to help regulate blood sugar levels. Regular physical activity is encouraged to improve insulin sensitivity, promote weight management, and enhance overall cardiovascular health. Additionally, monitoring blood sugar levels through self-testing or continuous glucose monitoring is crucial for adjusting treatment regimens and preventing complications.

The Role of Herbal Juicing in Diabetes Management

Dr. Barbara's holistic approach introduces herbal juicing as a complementary therapy to conventional diabetes management. Herbal juicing involves extracting the beneficial compounds from fresh herbs and vegetables by blending or juicing them into a concentrated liquid form. These juices are rich in vitamins, minerals, antioxidants, and bioactive compounds that possess various health-promoting properties, including anti-inflammatory, antioxidant, and hypoglycemic effects.

Herbs for Diabetes Management

Several herbs have shown promise in supporting diabetes management by helping to regulate blood sugar levels, improve insulin sensitivity, and mitigate complications associated with the condition. Some commonly used herbs in Dr. Barbara's approach include:

1. **Bitter Melon**: Bitter melon, also known as bitter gourd or Momordica charantia, is a tropical vine widely cultivated for its edible fruit, which has a distinctively bitter taste. Studies have suggested that bitter melon may help lower blood sugar levels by increasing insulin secretion, improving glucose utilization, and reducing insulin resistance.

2. **Fenugreek**: Fenugreek seeds contain soluble fiber and compounds like trigonelline and galactomannan, which have been shown to help lower blood sugar levels by delaying carbohydrate absorption and enhancing insulin action. Fenugreek may also improve lipid profiles and reduce the risk of cardiovascular complications in diabetes.

3. **Cinnamon**: Cinnamon is a popular spice derived from the bark of the Cinnamomum tree and is known for its sweet

and warm flavor. Research suggests that cinnamon may help improve insulin sensitivity, lower fasting blood sugar levels, and reduce postprandial glucose spikes in individuals with diabetes.

4. **Gymnema Sylvestre**: Gymnemasylvestre, also known as gurmar or "sugar destroyer," is an herb native to India and has been traditionally used in Ayurvedic medicine to support blood sugar control. Gymnemic acids found in the leaves of this plant may help reduce sugar cravings, enhance insulin secretion, and improve glucose utilization by cells.

5. **Turmeric**: Turmeric, a bright yellow spice derived from the Curcuma longa plant, contains curcumin, a potent antioxidant and anti-inflammatory compound. Studies have suggested that curcumin may help lower blood sugar levels, improve insulin sensitivity, and protect against diabetic complications by reducing oxidative stress and inflammation.

Preparing Herbal Juices

Dr. Barbara's approach emphasizes the importance of using fresh, organic herbs and vegetables to prepare herbal juices to maximize their therapeutic benefits. The process typically involves washing the ingredients thoroughly, removing any seeds or pits, and blending or juicing them into a smooth liquid. It's essential to consume the juice immediately to preserve its nutritional content and avoid oxidation. Additionally, combining different herbs and vegetables in various recipes can create flavorful and diverse options while providing a spectrum of health-promoting nutrients.

Incorporating Herbal Juices into Daily Routine

To reap the full benefits of herbal juicing in diabetes management, it's important to incorporate these juices into a balanced and individualized daily routine. Dr. Barbara recommends consuming herbal juices as part of a nutrient-rich diet that includes whole grains, lean proteins, healthy fats, and plenty of fruits and vegetables. Herbal juices can be enjoyed as a refreshing beverage between meals, as a component of smoothies or shakes, or as a base for soups and sauces. It's crucial to monitor blood sugar levels regularly and adjust medication or dietary intake accordingly to maintain optimal glycemic control.

Conclusion

Dr. Barbara's holistic approach to managing diabetes with herbal juicing offers a complementary strategy that harnesses the therapeutic properties of herbs and vegetables to support blood sugar regulation, improve insulin sensitivity, and enhance overall well-being. By incorporating fresh, organic ingredients into delicious and nutritious juices, individuals with diabetes can empower themselves to take an active role in their health and complement conventional treatment modalities with natural and holistic interventions. However, it's essential to consult with a healthcare professional before making any significant changes to your diabetes management plan and to monitor blood sugar levels regularly to ensure safety and efficacy.

CHAPTER TWO

Understanding Diabetes: Dr. Barbara's Insights into the Disease and Its Impact on Health

Dr. Barbara brings a unique perspective to understanding diabetes, a chronic metabolic disorder characterized by elevated levels of blood glucose (sugar). Her insights delve into the multifaceted nature of diabetes and its profound impact on overall health and well-being. By exploring the physiological mechanisms underlying the disease and its associated complications, Dr. Barbara sheds light on the importance of comprehensive management strategies that address not only blood sugar regulation but also other aspects of health affected by diabetes.

The Physiology of Diabetes

At the core of diabetes lies a disruption in the body's ability to regulate blood sugar levels effectively. Under normal circumstances, the pancreas produces insulin, a hormone responsible for facilitating the uptake of glucose into cells, where it is utilized for energy production or stored for future use. However, in individuals with diabetes, this intricate regulatory system is compromised, leading to either insufficient insulin production (Type 1 diabetes) or resistance to insulin action (Type 2 diabetes).

In Type 1 diabetes, the immune system mistakenly attacks and destroys the insulin-producing beta cells in the pancreas, resulting in an absolute deficiency of insulin. Without adequate insulin, glucose accumulates in the bloodstream, leading to hyperglycemia and depriving cells of the energy they need to function properly.

Type 2 diabetes, on the other hand, is characterized by insulin resistance, where cells become less responsive to the effects of insulin, necessitating higher insulin levels to maintain normal blood sugar levels. Over time, the pancreas may become unable to produce enough insulin to compensate for insulin resistance, leading to elevated blood glucose levels and the onset of diabetes.

Impact on Health and Well-being

The ramifications of uncontrolled diabetes extend far beyond elevated blood sugar levels. Diabetes affects nearly every system in the body and is associated with a myriad of complications that can significantly impact health and quality of life. Some of the most common complications of diabetes include:

1. **Cardiovascular Disease**: Diabetes increases the risk of developing cardiovascular conditions such as heart disease, stroke, and peripheral artery disease. Elevated blood sugar levels, along with other metabolic abnormalities associated with diabetes, contribute to the development of

atherosclerosis (hardening and narrowing of the arteries) and increase the likelihood of heart attacks and strokes.

2. **Neuropathy**: Chronic high blood sugar levels can damage the nerves throughout the body, leading to diabetic neuropathy. Symptoms may include numbness, tingling, burning sensations, and weakness, particularly in the extremities. Diabetic neuropathy can impair sensation and motor function, increasing the risk of injuries and infections, particularly in the feet.

3. **Nephropathy**: Diabetes is a leading cause of kidney disease, known as diabetic nephropathy. Persistent high blood sugar levels can damage the small blood vessels in the kidneys, impairing their ability to filter waste products from the blood effectively. Over time, diabetic nephropathy can progress to chronic kidney disease and ultimately, kidney failure, necessitating dialysis or kidney transplantation.

4. **Retinopathy**: Diabetes is a significant risk factor for vision loss and blindness due to diabetic retinopathy, a condition characterized by damage to the blood vessels in the retina. Elevated blood sugar levels cause the blood vessels in the retina to become weak and leaky, leading to retinal swelling, hemorrhage, and ultimately, vision impairment or blindness if left untreated.

5. **Foot Complications**: Diabetes increases the risk of foot problems, including foot ulcers, infections, and Charcot arthropathy (joint damage caused by nerve damage). Peripheral neuropathy, poor circulation, and impaired wound healing contribute to the development of foot complications, which can lead to serious infections and, in severe cases, amputation.

Dr. Barbara's Approach to Diabetes Management

Dr. Barbara recognizes the complex interplay between diabetes and overall health and emphasizes a holistic approach to diabetes management that addresses not only blood sugar regulation but also other aspects of health affected by the disease. Her approach encompasses a comprehensive strategy that integrates dietary modifications, regular physical activity, stress management, adequate sleep, and, importantly, herbal juicing as a natural adjunct to conventional treatment modalities.

By focusing on whole foods, particularly plant-based foods rich in fiber, vitamins, minerals, and antioxidants, Dr. Barbara promotes optimal nutrition to support blood sugar control, cardiovascular health, and overall well-being. Regular physical activity is encouraged to improve insulin sensitivity, promote weight management, and reduce the risk of cardiovascular complications associated with diabetes.

Incorporating stress management techniques such as mindfulness meditation, deep breathing exercises, and yoga can help mitigate the physiological and psychological effects of stress, which can exacerbate blood sugar fluctuations in individuals with diabetes. Adequate sleep is also essential for maintaining hormonal balance, supporting immune function, and optimizing metabolic health.

Herbal juicing is a key component of Dr. Barbara's holistic approach to diabetes management, harnessing the therapeutic properties of herbs and vegetables to support blood sugar regulation, improve insulin sensitivity, and enhance overall health. By incorporating fresh, organic ingredients into delicious and nutritious juices, individuals with diabetes can complement conventional treatment modalities with natural and holistic interventions that empower them to take control of their health and well-being.

In conclusion, Dr. Barbara's insights into diabetes underscore the importance of understanding the multifaceted nature of the disease and its profound impact on health and well-being. By adopting a holistic approach to diabetes management that addresses not only blood sugar regulation but also other aspects of health affected by the disease, individuals can optimize their outcomes and enhance their quality of life. Through dietary modifications, regular physical activity, stress management, adequate sleep, and herbal juicing, individuals can empower themselves to take an active role in managing their diabetes and promoting long-term health and vitality.

CHAPTER THREE

The Healing Power of Herbal Juicing: How Fresh Juices Can Support Diabetes Control

Herbal juicing has emerged as a popular and effective strategy for managing diabetes, offering a natural approach that harnesses the healing power of herbs and vegetables to support blood sugar control and overall health. Dr. Barbara's holistic approach emphasizes the therapeutic benefits of fresh juices, highlighting their potential to complement conventional treatment modalities and enhance diabetes management. By exploring the mechanisms underlying the healing properties of herbal juices and their specific effects on blood sugar regulation, this article delves into the role of juicing in supporting diabetes control and promoting well-being.

Understanding Herbal Juicing

Herbal juicing involves extracting the beneficial compounds from fresh herbs and vegetables by blending or juicing them into a concentrated liquid form. These juices are rich in vitamins, minerals, antioxidants, and phytochemicals, which possess various health-promoting properties. Unlike processed juices or sugary beverages, which can contribute to blood sugar spikes and insulin resistance, fresh herbal juices offer a nutrient-dense and low-glycemic option that supports blood sugar regulation and overall health.

Herbs and Vegetables for Diabetes Control

Several herbs and vegetables have been shown to have beneficial effects on blood sugar control and insulin sensitivity, making them ideal ingredients for herbal juices targeted at managing diabetes. Some key herbs and vegetables used in Dr. Barbara's approach include:

1. **Bitter Melon**: Bitter melon is renowned for its hypoglycemic properties, attributed to compounds like charantin, polypeptide-p, and vicine. These compounds help lower blood sugar levels by increasing insulin secretion, improving glucose uptake by cells, and reducing insulin resistance. Incorporating bitter melon juice into the diet can support blood sugar control and enhance insulin sensitivity in individuals with diabetes.

2. **Fenugreek**: Fenugreek seeds contain soluble fiber and compounds like trigonelline and galactomannan, which help lower blood sugar levels by delaying carbohydrate absorption and improving insulin sensitivity. Fenugreek juice can be a valuable addition to diabetes management strategies, helping stabilize blood sugar levels and reduce postprandial glucose spikes.

3. **Cinnamon**: Cinnamon is prized for its sweet and warm flavor and its potential to improve blood sugar control in individuals with diabetes. Active compounds like

cinnamaldehyde and cinnamic acid help enhance insulin sensitivity, reduce insulin resistance, and lower fasting blood sugar levels. Adding cinnamon juice to beverages or recipes can impart both flavor and health benefits for individuals with diabetes.

4. **Gymnema Sylvestre**: Gymnemasylvestre, also known as "sugar destroyer," has a long history of use in traditional medicine for its ability to support blood sugar regulation. Gymnemic acids found in the leaves of this plant help reduce sugar cravings, inhibit glucose absorption in the intestines, and stimulate insulin secretion from pancreatic beta cells. Incorporating gymnemasylvestre juice into the diet can help individuals with diabetes manage their blood sugar levels more effectively.

5. **Turmeric**: Turmeric contains curcumin, a potent antioxidant and anti-inflammatory compound that offers various health benefits, including improved blood sugar control. Curcumin helps lower blood sugar levels, enhance insulin sensitivity, and reduce inflammation, making it a valuable addition to herbal juices for diabetes management.

Mechanisms of Action

The therapeutic effects of herbal juices in diabetes control stem from their diverse array of bioactive compounds, which target multiple pathways involved in blood sugar regulation and insulin sensitivity. These mechanisms include:

1. **Increasing Insulin Secretion**: Certain herbs like bitter melon and gymnemasylvestre stimulate insulin secretion from pancreatic beta cells, helping lower blood sugar levels by promoting the uptake of glucose into cells.

2. **Improving Glucose Utilization**: Compounds like fenugreek and cinnamon enhance glucose uptake by cells, improving insulin sensitivity and reducing insulin resistance.

3. **Inhibiting Glucose Absorption**: Some herbs, such as gymnemasylvestre, inhibit glucose absorption in the intestines, reducing postprandial blood sugar spikes and promoting more stable blood sugar levels.

4. **Reducing Sugar Cravings**: Gymnemasylvestre contains compounds that suppress sweet cravings, helping individuals with diabetes control their appetite and reduce their intake of sugary foods and beverages.

5. **Protecting Pancreatic Beta Cells**: Certain herbs possess antioxidant and anti-inflammatory properties that protect pancreatic beta cells from oxidative stress and inflammation, preserving their function and promoting insulin secretion.

Incorporating Herbal Juices into Diabetes Management

Dr. Barbara's approach emphasizes the importance of incorporating herbal juices into a comprehensive diabetes management plan that includes dietary modifications, regular physical activity, stress management, and medication as needed. Herbal juices can be enjoyed as part of a balanced and nutrient-rich diet, providing a refreshing and flavorful way to support blood sugar control and overall health.

To incorporate herbal juices into diabetes management effectively, individuals should:

1. **Choose Fresh, Organic Ingredients**: Opt for fresh, organic herbs and vegetables whenever possible to maximize their nutritional content and minimize exposure to pesticides and other contaminants.

2. **Experiment with Different Combinations**: Explore a variety of herbs and vegetables to create flavorful and diverse juice recipes that suit individual tastes and preferences. Combining different ingredients can also provide a broader spectrum of health benefits.

3. **Monitor Blood Sugar Levels**: Regularly monitor blood sugar levels to assess the impact of herbal juices on glycemic control and adjust dietary intake or medication as needed. It's essential to work closely with a healthcare provider to ensure safe and effective diabetes management.

4. **Integrate Juicing into Daily Routine**: Incorporate herbal juices into daily meals and snacks as part of a balanced and individualized diabetes management plan. Herbal juices can be enjoyed as a refreshing beverage, incorporated into smoothies or shakes, or used as a base for soups and sauces.

5. **Be Mindful of Portion Sizes**: While herbal juices offer numerous health benefits, they still contain calories and carbohydrates that can affect blood sugar levels. Be mindful of portion sizes and monitor the overall carbohydrate content of meals and snacks to maintain optimal glycemic control.

Conclusion

Herbal juicing offers a natural and effective approach to supporting diabetes control and promoting overall health and well-being. By harnessing the healing power of herbs and vegetables, individuals with diabetes can complement conventional treatment modalities with fresh and nutrient-rich juices that support blood sugar regulation, improve insulin sensitivity, and reduce the risk of complications associated with the disease. Through experimentation with different ingredients, mindful monitoring of blood sugar levels, and integration into daily routines, herbal juices can empower individuals with diabetes to take an active role in managing their health and optimizing their outcomes.

CHAPTER FOUR

Preparing for Your Juicing Journey: Setting Goals and Gathering Ingredients

Embarking on a juicing journey can be an exciting and rewarding endeavor, especially when aiming to manage diabetes through holistic approaches like herbal juicing. Before diving into juicing, it's crucial to set clear goals and gather the right ingredients to ensure a successful and sustainable experience. In this guide, we'll explore the importance of goal setting, offer tips for selecting ingredients, and provide guidance on how to prepare for your juicing journey effectively.

Setting Clear Goals

Setting clear and realistic goals is essential for any health-related endeavor, including juicing for diabetes management. When setting your goals, consider the following factors:

1. **Blood Sugar Control**: Determine your target blood sugar range and establish specific goals for achieving and maintaining optimal blood sugar levels throughout the day.

2. **Weight Management**: If weight management is a priority, set goals for achieving a healthy weight or maintaining weight loss through juicing and dietary modifications.

3. **Nutritional Support**: Identify specific nutritional needs related to diabetes management, such as increasing intake

of certain vitamins, minerals, and antioxidants, and set goals for meeting these needs through juicing.

4. **Energy and Well-being**: Consider how juicing can enhance your overall energy levels, mood, and sense of well-being, and set goals for improving these aspects of your health.

5. **Long-Term Sustainability**: Aim to set goals that are sustainable over the long term, focusing on lifestyle changes that you can maintain consistently to support your health and well-being.

By setting clear and achievable goals, you can stay motivated and focused on your juicing journey, increasing the likelihood of success in managing diabetes and improving your overall health.

Selecting Ingredients for Juicing

Selecting the right ingredients is crucial for creating delicious and nutritious juices that support your diabetes management goals. When choosing ingredients for juicing, consider the following tips:

1. **Focus on Fresh, Whole Foods**: Opt for fresh, organic fruits, vegetables, and herbs whenever possible to maximize their nutritional content and minimize exposure to pesticides and other contaminants.

2. **Choose Low-Glycemic Ingredients**: Select fruits and vegetables with a low glycemic index (GI) to help minimize blood sugar spikes. Examples of low-GI fruits and vegetables

include leafy greens, cucumbers, celery, berries, and citrus fruits.

3. **Incorporate Diabetes-Friendly Herbs**: Include herbs and spices with known benefits for diabetes management, such as bitter melon, fenugreek, cinnamon, turmeric, and ginger, to enhance the nutritional profile and therapeutic properties of your juices.

4. **Balance Flavors and Textures**: Experiment with different combinations of fruits, vegetables, and herbs to create flavorful and balanced juices. Consider combining sweet, tart, and savory ingredients to achieve a harmonious blend of flavors and textures.

5. **Variety is Key**: Aim to include a variety of ingredients in your juices to ensure a diverse array of nutrients and phytochemicals. Rotate your ingredient choices regularly to prevent boredom and maximize nutritional benefits.

6. **Mindful Portion Control**: Be mindful of portion sizes when juicing fruits, as they can contribute to higher sugar content and calorie intake. Focus on incorporating more vegetables than fruits into your juices to help minimize sugar content while still enjoying delicious flavors.

Preparing Your Juicing Station

Once you've selected your ingredients, it's time to prepare your juicing station to streamline the juicing process and make it more convenient and enjoyable. Consider the following steps:

1. **Organize Your Ingredients**: Wash, peel, and chop your fruits, vegetables, and herbs in advance to save time during juicing. Store prepped ingredients in airtight containers or bags in the refrigerator until ready to use.

2. **Set Up Your Juicer**: Ensure your juicer is clean and assembled according to the manufacturer's instructions. Place it on a stable surface near a power source and have a pitcher or container ready to collect the juice.

3. **Gather Necessary Tools**: Gather essential tools and accessories, such as a cutting board, knife, citrus juicer, measuring cups, and spoons, to facilitate the juicing process and minimize messes.

4. **Create a Juicing Schedule**: Establish a juicing schedule that fits into your daily routine and allows you to incorporate fresh juices into your meals and snacks seamlessly. Consider juicing in the morning for a refreshing start to the day or preparing juices in advance for on-the-go convenience.

5. **Clean as You Go**: Clean your juicer and workspace promptly after juicing to prevent residue buildup and make cleanup

easier. Rinse juicer components with warm, soapy water and wipe down countertops and surfaces with a damp cloth.

Conclusion

Preparing for your juicing journey involves setting clear goals, selecting the right ingredients, and organizing your juicing station to streamline the process and maximize convenience. By establishing realistic goals, choosing fresh and nutritious ingredients, and creating a well-equipped juicing station, you can set yourself up for success in managing diabetes through herbal juicing. With dedication, creativity, and mindful preparation, you can embark on a fulfilling and health-enhancing juicing journey that supports your diabetes management goals and promotes overall well-being.

CHAPTER FIVE

Selecting the Right Herbs: Dr. Barbara's Recommended Ingredients for Juicing to Manage Diabetes

Dr. Barbara's holistic approach to managing diabetes through herbal juicing emphasizes the therapeutic benefits of specific herbs known for their ability to support blood sugar regulation, improve insulin sensitivity, and enhance overall health. By incorporating these carefully selected herbs into your juicing routine, you can create delicious and nutritious juices that complement conventional treatment modalities and promote well-being. In this guide, we'll explore Dr. Barbara's recommended herbs for juicing to manage diabetes and their specific benefits for supporting your health goals.

Bitter Melon

Bitter melon (Momordica charantia) is a tropical vine widely cultivated for its edible fruit, which has a distinctively bitter taste. It is prized for its potent hypoglycemic properties and has been used traditionally in various cultures to manage diabetes. Bitter melon contains compounds like charantin, polypeptide-p, and vicine, which help lower blood sugar levels by increasing insulin secretion, improving glucose uptake by cells, and reducing insulin resistance. Incorporating bitter melon juice into your juicing routine can support blood sugar regulation and enhance insulin sensitivity in individuals with diabetes.

Fenugreek

Fenugreek (Trigonella foenum-graecum) seeds are rich in soluble fiber and bioactive compounds like trigonelline and galactomannan, which have been shown to help lower blood sugar levels and improve insulin sensitivity. Fenugreek seeds also contain amino acids that stimulate insulin secretion and inhibit the breakdown of carbohydrates into glucose. Adding fenugreek juice to your juicing repertoire can help stabilize blood sugar levels, reduce postprandial glucose spikes, and support overall diabetes management.

Cinnamon

Cinnamon is a popular spice derived from the bark of the Cinnamomum tree and is prized for its sweet and warm flavor. It contains active compounds like cinnamaldehyde and cinnamic acid, which have been shown to improve insulin sensitivity, reduce insulin resistance, and lower fasting blood sugar levels in individuals with diabetes. Cinnamon also has antioxidant and anti-inflammatory properties that can help protect against diabetic complications. Incorporating cinnamon juice into your juicing routine can enhance the flavor and health benefits of your juices while supporting blood sugar control.

Gymnema Sylvestre

Gymnemasylvestre, also known as "sugar destroyer," is an herb native to India and has a long history of use in Ayurvedic medicine for its ability to support blood sugar regulation. Gymnemic acids found in the leaves of this plant help reduce sugar cravings, inhibit glucose absorption in the intestines, and stimulate insulin secretion from pancreatic beta cells. Gymnemasylvestre juice can be a valuable addition to your juicing routine, helping you manage your blood sugar levels more effectively and reduce the risk of diabetic complications.

Turmeric

Turmeric (Curcuma longa) is a bright yellow spice prized for its potent antioxidant and anti-inflammatory properties. It contains curcumin, a bioactive compound that has been shown to help lower blood sugar levels, improve insulin sensitivity, and reduce inflammation in individuals with diabetes. Turmeric also supports cardiovascular health and may help prevent diabetic complications. Incorporating turmeric juice into your juicing routine can add a vibrant color and robust flavor to your juices while providing numerous health benefits for managing diabetes.

Ginger

Ginger (Zingiber officinale) is a versatile herb known for its spicy flavor and medicinal properties. It contains bioactive compounds like gingerol and shogaol, which have been shown to help improve insulin sensitivity, reduce inflammation, and lower blood sugar levels in individuals with diabetes. Ginger also supports digestion, reduces nausea, and may help prevent diabetic complications like neuropathy and nephropathy. Adding ginger juice to your juicing repertoire can enhance the flavor and health benefits of your juices while supporting your diabetes management goals.

Conclusion

Incorporating Dr. Barbara's recommended herbs into your juicing routine can support blood sugar regulation, improve insulin sensitivity, and enhance overall health in individuals with diabetes. By selecting fresh, organic herbs and incorporating them into delicious and nutritious juices, you can complement conventional treatment modalities and empower yourself to take an active role in managing your diabetes. Experiment with different combinations of herbs, fruits, and vegetables to create flavorful and diverse juices that support your health goals and promote well-being. With dedication, creativity, and mindful selection of ingredients, you can embark on a fulfilling and health-enhancing juicing journey that supports your diabetes management journey and enhances your quality of life.

CHAPTER SIX

Crafting Healing Recipes: Juices Designed to Stabilize Blood Sugar Levels and Promote Wellness

Crafting healing juices designed to stabilize blood sugar levels and promote overall wellness requires careful selection of ingredients and thoughtful combination of flavors. Dr. Barbara's holistic approach emphasizes the use of fresh, organic herbs, vegetables, and fruits known for their therapeutic properties in managing diabetes and supporting health goals. By incorporating these ingredients into delicious and nutrient-rich juices, you can create flavorful beverages that complement conventional treatment modalities and enhance your well-being. In this guide, we'll explore several healing juice recipes tailored to stabilize blood sugar levels and promote wellness.

1. Bitter Green Elixir

Bitter greens, such as kale, spinach, and bitter melon, are rich in antioxidants and phytonutrients that support blood sugar regulation and promote overall health.

- 2 cups kale leaves
- 1 cup spinach leaves
- 1/2 medium bitter melon, seeds removed

- 1 green apple, cored
- 1/2 cucumber
- 1-inch piece of ginger
- Juice of 1 lemon

Instructions:

1. Wash all ingredients thoroughly.
2. Chop the kale, spinach, bitter melon, apple, and cucumber into smaller pieces to fit into your juicer.
3. Juice all the ingredients, including the ginger and lemon, according to your juicer's instructions.
4. Stir the juice well to combine the flavors.
5. Serve immediately over ice, if desired.

2. Spiced Citrus Delight

Cinnamon and turmeric add warmth and depth of flavor to this citrus-infused juice, while ginger provides additional anti-inflammatory and blood sugar-regulating properties.

- 2 oranges, peeled
- 1 grapefruit, peeled
- 1/2 lemon, peeled

- 1-inch piece of ginger
- 1/2 teaspoon ground cinnamon
- 1/4 teaspoon ground turmeric

Instructions:

1. Peel the oranges, grapefruit, and lemon, removing any seeds.
2. Cut the ginger into smaller pieces.
3. Juice the oranges, grapefruit, lemon, and ginger in your juicer.
4. Stir in the ground cinnamon and turmeric.
5. Mix well to combine the spices with the juice.
6. Serve immediately for optimal flavor and nutritional benefits.

3. Green Goddess Detox

This refreshing green juice is packed with detoxifying and blood sugar-stabilizing ingredients, including celery, cucumber, and parsley.

- 4 celery stalks
- 1 cucumber
- 1 cup parsley leaves

- 1 green apple, cored
- 1/2 lemon, peeled
- 1-inch piece of ginger

Instructions:

1. Wash all ingredients thoroughly.
2. Chop the celery, cucumber, parsley, apple, and lemon into smaller pieces.
3. Juice all the ingredients, including the ginger, in your juicer.
4. Stir the juice well to combine the flavors.
5. Serve immediately over ice, if desired, for a refreshing and revitalizing drink.

4. Berry Blast Antioxidant Booster

Berries are rich in antioxidants and fiber, making them excellent choices for stabilizing blood sugar levels and promoting overall health.

- 1 cup mixed berries (such as strawberries, blueberries, and raspberries)
- 1 small beet, peeled
- 1 carrot, peeled
- 1/2 cucumber

- 1-inch piece of ginger
- Juice of 1/2 lemon

Instructions:

1. Wash all ingredients thoroughly.
2. Cut the beet, carrot, cucumber, and ginger into smaller pieces.
3. Juice all the ingredients, including the mixed berries and lemon juice, in your juicer.
4. Stir the juice well to combine the flavors.
5. Serve immediately for a refreshing and antioxidant-rich beverage.

5. Turmeric Spice Soother

This warming and soothing juice blend combine the anti-inflammatory properties of turmeric with the digestive benefits of ginger and lemon.

- 2 large carrots, peeled
- 1 small orange, peeled
- 1-inch piece of turmeric root
- 1-inch piece of ginger
- Juice of 1/2 lemon

- Pinch of black pepper (to enhance the absorption of turmeric)

Instructions:

1. Wash all ingredients thoroughly.
2. Cut the carrots, orange, turmeric, and ginger into smaller pieces.
3. Juice all the ingredients, including the lemon juice and black pepper, in your juicer.
4. Stir the juice well to combine the flavors.
5. Serve immediately for a comforting and immune-boosting drink.

Conclusion

Crafting healing juice recipes designed to stabilize blood sugar levels and promote overall wellness involves selecting the right ingredients and combining them thoughtfully to maximize their therapeutic benefits. By incorporating fresh, organic herbs, vegetables, and fruits known for their blood sugar-regulating properties into your juices, you can create flavorful and nutrient-rich beverages that support your health goals. Experiment with different combinations of ingredients and flavors to find the recipes that work best for you, and enjoy the nourishing benefits of juicing as part of your diabetes management and wellness routine.

CHAPTER SEVEN

Incorporating Additional Nutrients: Enhancing the Nutritional Value of Your Juices for Diabetes Management

Enhancing the nutritional value of your juices for diabetes management involves incorporating additional nutrients that support blood sugar regulation, promote overall health, and provide essential vitamins, minerals, and antioxidants. By selecting nutrient-dense ingredients and incorporating them into your juicing routine, you can create delicious and balanced beverages that complement your diabetes management plan. In this guide, we'll explore various ways to enhance the nutritional value of your juices and optimize their benefits for diabetes management.

1. Add Leafy Greens

Leafy greens, such as kale, spinach, and Swiss chard, are nutritional powerhouses rich in vitamins, minerals, and antioxidants. They are low in calories and carbohydrates, making them ideal ingredients for managing blood sugar levels. Incorporating leafy greens into your juices adds essential nutrients like vitamin K, vitamin C, folate, and magnesium, which support overall health and well-being.

2. Include Fiber-Rich Ingredients

Fiber plays a crucial role in diabetes management by slowing down the absorption of sugar into the bloodstream and promoting satiety. Adding fiber-rich ingredients like celery, cucumber, and flaxseeds to your juices can help stabilize blood sugar levels and improve digestive health. These ingredients also contribute to a feeling of fullness, which can aid in weight management and reduce the risk of overeating.

3. Incorporate Protein Sources

Protein is essential for maintaining muscle mass, supporting metabolism, and promoting satiety. Including protein sources like Greek yogurt, tofu, or plant-based protein powders in your juices can help balance blood sugar levels and prevent spikes in insulin production. Protein-rich ingredients also provide amino acids that support muscle repair and recovery, particularly important for individuals with diabetes who may experience muscle weakness or loss.

4. Add Healthy Fats

Healthy fats, such as avocados, nuts, and seeds, provide essential fatty acids that support heart health, brain function, and overall well-being. Incorporating sources of healthy fats into your juices, such as avocado or flaxseed oil, can help stabilize blood sugar levels and enhance nutrient absorption. These ingredients also contribute to a creamy texture and rich flavor, making your juices more satisfying and enjoyable to consume.

5. Include Blood Sugar-Stabilizing Spices

Certain spices have been shown to have blood sugar-stabilizing properties and can be valuable additions to your juices. Cinnamon, turmeric, and ginger are examples of spices that help improve insulin sensitivity, reduce inflammation, and promote overall health. Incorporating these spices into your juices adds depth of flavor and enhances their therapeutic benefits for diabetes management.

6. Choose Low-Glycemic Fruits

While fruits contain natural sugars, some have a lower glycemic index (GI) than others, meaning they have less of an impact on blood sugar levels. Opt for low-glycemic fruits like berries, apples, and citrus fruits when creating juices for diabetes management. These fruits provide essential vitamins, minerals, and antioxidants without causing significant spikes in blood sugar.

7. Balance Your Ingredients

When crafting your juices, aim for a balanced combination of fruits, vegetables, protein, fiber, and healthy fats to create a satisfying and nutritious beverage. Experiment with different ingredient combinations to find the right balance that works for your taste preferences and nutritional needs. Pay attention to portion sizes and monitor your blood sugar levels to ensure that your juices are supporting your diabetes management goals effectively.

Conclusion

Enhancing the nutritional value of your juices for diabetes management involves incorporating nutrient-dense ingredients that support blood sugar regulation, promote overall health, and provide essential vitamins, minerals, and antioxidants. By adding leafy greens, fiber-rich ingredients, protein sources, healthy fats, blood sugar-stabilizing spices, and low-glycemic fruits to your juices, you can create delicious and balanced beverages that complement your diabetes management plan. Experiment with different ingredient combinations, and enjoy the nourishing benefits of nutrient-rich juices as part of your daily routine.

CHAPTER EIGHT

Navigating Challenges: Tips for Adjusting to Juicing and Managing Blood Sugar Fluctuations

Embarking on a juicing journey to manage diabetes can bring numerous benefits, but it may also present challenges, especially when adjusting to new dietary habits and managing blood sugar fluctuations. By understanding common challenges and implementing strategies to overcome them, you can navigate the transition to juicing more effectively and achieve better control over your diabetes. In this guide, we'll explore tips for adjusting to juicing and managing blood sugar fluctuations to support your overall health and well-being.

1. Monitor Blood Sugar Levels Regularly

One of the most crucial aspects of managing diabetes while juicing is monitoring your blood sugar levels regularly. Keep track of your blood sugar readings before and after consuming juices to understand how different ingredients affect your glucose levels. This information can help you make informed decisions about ingredient choices, portion sizes, and timing to optimize blood sugar control.

2. Experiment with Ingredient Combinations

Every individual's response to juicing ingredients may vary, so it's essential to experiment with different combinations to find what works best for you. Pay attention to how specific fruits, vegetables, herbs, and spices affect your blood sugar levels and adjust your recipes accordingly. Focus on incorporating low-glycemic ingredients and balancing carbohydrates with protein, fiber, and healthy fats to minimize blood sugar fluctuations.

3. Limit High-Glycemic Ingredients

While fruits are nutritious and delicious, some may have a higher glycemic index (GI) and can cause rapid spikes in blood sugar levels. Limit high-glycemic fruits like pineapple, watermelon, and ripe bananas in your juices and opt for lower-glycemic options such as berries, apples, and citrus fruits. Balancing high-glycemic ingredients with fiber-rich vegetables and protein sources can help mitigate their impact on blood sugar.

4. Include Protein and Healthy Fats

Incorporating protein and healthy fats into your juices can help slow down the absorption of carbohydrates and stabilize blood sugar levels. Add ingredients like Greek yogurt, tofu, avocado, nuts, and seeds to your juices to provide satiety and prevent rapid blood sugar spikes. Protein and healthy fats also contribute to a balanced diet and promote overall well-being.

5. Mindful Portion Control

Even though juices are nutritious, they still contain calories and carbohydrates that can affect blood sugar levels. Practice mindful portion control when consuming juices and avoid overindulging, especially if you're trying to manage your weight or blood sugar. Stick to recommended serving sizes and monitor your portion sizes to maintain optimal blood sugar control.

6. Stay Hydrated

Hydration is essential for overall health and can also help regulate blood sugar levels. Drink plenty of water throughout the day, especially when consuming juices, to stay hydrated and support proper digestion and nutrient absorption. Avoid sugary beverages and opt for water, herbal teas, or infused water to quench your thirst without adding extra calories or carbohydrates.

7. Be Patient and Persistent

Adjusting to juicing and managing blood sugar fluctuations may take time and patience. Be patient with yourself as you explore different recipes, ingredients, and strategies to optimize your diabetes management. Stay persistent in your efforts to maintain a healthy lifestyle, and don't be discouraged by setbacks or challenges along the way. With dedication and perseverance, you can overcome obstacles and achieve better control over your diabetes.

8. Consult with a Healthcare Professional

If you're unsure about how juicing may impact your diabetes management or if you have specific concerns or questions, consult with a healthcare professional, such as a registered dietitian or diabetes educator. They can provide personalized guidance, tailored recommendations, and support to help you navigate the complexities of juicing and diabetes management effectively.

Conclusion

Adjusting to juicing and managing blood sugar fluctuations requires patience, experimentation, and proactive monitoring. By implementing strategies such as monitoring blood sugar levels regularly, experimenting with ingredient combinations, limiting high-glycemic ingredients, including protein and healthy fats, practicing mindful portion control, staying hydrated, and seeking guidance from healthcare professionals, you can navigate the challenges of juicing and diabetes management successfully. With dedication, mindfulness, and support, you can harness the benefits of juicing to improve your overall health and well-being while effectively managing your diabetes.

CHAPTER NINE

Success Stories: Real-Life Accounts of Individuals Who Have Improved Their Diabetes Through Herbal Juicing

Real-life success stories offer inspiring examples of how individuals have transformed their health and improved their diabetes management through herbal juicing. By incorporating fresh, nutrient-rich juices into their daily routines, these individuals have experienced significant improvements in blood sugar control, weight management, and overall well-being. In this compilation of success stories, we'll explore firsthand accounts of individuals who have successfully managed their diabetes through herbal juicing and achieved remarkable results.

Case Study 1: Sarah's Journey to Better Blood Sugar Control

Sarah, a 45-year-old woman diagnosed with type 2 diabetes, struggled with fluctuating blood sugar levels despite medication and dietary modifications. Seeking a natural approach to managing her condition, Sarah began incorporating herbal juicing into her daily routine. She experimented with various combinations of herbs, vegetables, and fruits known for their blood sugar-regulating properties, such as bitter melon, fenugreek, and turmeric.

Within weeks of starting her juicing regimen, Sarah noticed significant improvements in her blood sugar levels. Her fasting blood sugar readings became more stable, and she experienced fewer spikes and crashes throughout the day. Sarah also noticed an increase in energy levels, improved digestion, and better overall mood. Encouraged by her progress, Sarah continued with her juicing routine and eventually reduced her reliance on diabetes medication under the guidance of her healthcare provider.

Today, Sarah enjoys vibrant health and vitality, thanks to her commitment to herbal juicing and holistic wellness practices. She credits juicing with empowering her to take control of her diabetes and transform her health from the inside out.

Case Study 2: John's Weight Loss Journey with Juicing

John, a 55-year-old man with type 2 diabetes and obesity, struggled to manage his weight and blood sugar levels despite years of conventional treatment. Frustrated by his lack of progress, John decided to explore alternative approaches to diabetes management, including herbal juicing. He began incorporating fresh juices made from a combination of leafy greens, citrus fruits, and herbs into his daily routine.

As John embraced his juicing journey, he noticed gradual but significant changes in his health and well-being. He experienced weight loss, improved energy levels, and better blood sugar control. By replacing sugary snacks and processed foods with nutrient-dense juices, John was able to curb his cravings, reduce his calorie intake, and shed excess pounds.

Over time, John's diabetes symptoms improved, and he was able to reduce his reliance on medication. His healthcare provider was impressed by his progress and encouraged him to continue with his juicing routine as part of his diabetes management plan. Today, John enjoys a healthier lifestyle, improved self-confidence, and a renewed sense of vitality, all thanks to the power of herbal juicing.

Case Study 3: Maria's Journey to Diabetes Remission

Maria, a 50-year-old woman with type 2 diabetes, faced numerous health challenges, including obesity, high blood pressure, and insulin resistance. Determined to reclaim her health and reverse her diabetes diagnosis, Maria embarked on a holistic wellness journey that included herbal juicing as a central component. She focused on incorporating a variety of fresh, organic juices made from ingredients like bitter melon, fenugreek, spinach, and berries into her daily diet.

As Maria committed herself to her juicing routine, she experienced dramatic improvements in her health and well-being. Her blood sugar levels normalized, and she was able to reduce her reliance on diabetes medication gradually. Maria also lost weight, improved her cardiovascular health, and experienced increased vitality and mental clarity.

With the support of her healthcare team, Maria continued her juicing regimen and embraced other lifestyle modifications, such as regular exercise and stress management techniques. Through her dedication and perseverance, Maria achieved remission from diabetes and transformed her health in profound ways.

Conclusion

These real-life success stories demonstrate the transformative power of herbal juicing in managing diabetes and improving overall health and well-being. Through commitment, experimentation, and a willingness to embrace holistic approaches to wellness, individuals like Sarah, John, and Maria have achieved remarkable results and reclaimed their vitality. Their stories inspire hope and serve as reminders of the potential for positive change through natural interventions like herbal juicing. By harnessing the healing power of fresh, nutrient-rich juices, individuals with diabetes can take control of their health and embark on a journey toward greater vitality and well-being.

CHAPTER TEN

Beyond Juicing: Integrating Dr. Barbara's Principles for Long-Term Diabetes Management and Overall Health

Dr. Barbara's holistic approach to diabetes management extends beyond juicing to encompass a comprehensive wellness philosophy aimed at promoting long-term health and vitality. By integrating Dr. Barbara's principles into your lifestyle, you can enhance diabetes management, improve overall well-being, and cultivate habits that support lasting health benefits. In this guide, we'll explore key principles derived from Dr. Barbara's approach and discuss strategies for integrating them into your daily life for sustained diabetes management and optimal health.

1. Nutrient-Dense Diet

A cornerstone of Dr. Barbara's approach is the emphasis on a nutrient-dense diet rich in fresh fruits, vegetables, whole grains, lean proteins, and healthy fats. Beyond juicing, focus on incorporating a variety of whole foods into your meals and snacks to provide essential nutrients, fiber, and antioxidants that support blood sugar regulation, cardiovascular health, and overall well-being. Opt for minimally processed foods, and prioritize plant-based sources of protein and healthy fats to promote optimal health.

2. Regular Physical Activity

Physical activity plays a crucial role in diabetes management by improving insulin sensitivity, supporting weight management, and enhancing cardiovascular health. Integrate regular exercise into your routine, aiming for a combination of aerobic activities, strength training, and flexibility exercises. Find activities you enjoy and make them a priority, whether it's walking, swimming, cycling, yoga, or dancing. Aim for at least 150 minutes of moderate-intensity exercise per week, supplemented with strength training exercises two to three times per week.

3. Stress Management and Mindfulness

Chronic stress can exacerbate diabetes symptoms and negatively impact overall health. Incorporate stress management techniques such as mindfulness meditation, deep breathing exercises, yoga, tai chi, or progressive muscle relaxation into your daily routine. Cultivate practices that promote relaxation, self-awareness, and emotional well-being to reduce stress levels and enhance resilience in the face of life's challenges.

4. Adequate Sleep

Quality sleep is essential for diabetes management and overall health. Aim for seven to nine hours of uninterrupted sleep each night to support optimal blood sugar control, hormone regulation, and immune function. Establish a relaxing bedtime routine, create a comfortable sleep environment, and prioritize sleep hygiene practices such as limiting screen time before bed, avoiding caffeine and alcohol close to bedtime, and maintaining a consistent sleep schedule.

5. Regular Monitoring and Healthcare

Stay proactive in managing your diabetes by regularly monitoring your blood sugar levels, tracking your dietary intake and physical activity, and attending regular healthcare appointments. Work closely with your healthcare team, including your primary care physician, endocrinologist, registered dietitian, and diabetes educator, to develop a personalized diabetes management plan tailored to your individual needs and goals. Be open and honest about your challenges and concerns, and collaborate with your healthcare providers to optimize your treatment plan and support your overall health and well-being.

6. Community and Support

Seek support from family, friends, and peers who understand and support your journey with diabetes. Join diabetes support groups, participate in online forums, or engage in community events and activities that promote diabetes awareness and education. Surround yourself with a supportive network of individuals who can offer encouragement, advice, and understanding as you navigate the challenges and triumphs of living with diabetes.

Conclusion

Integrating Dr. Barbara's principles into your lifestyle goes beyond juicing to encompass a holistic approach to diabetes management and overall health. By prioritizing a nutrient-dense diet, regular physical activity, stress management, adequate sleep, regular monitoring and healthcare, and community support, you can cultivate habits that support long-term well-being and empower yourself to live well with diabetes. Embrace these principles as guiding principles for sustainable health and vitality, and commit to making gradual, sustainable changes that promote optimal health and wellness for years to come.

Sarsaparilla:

Definition: Sarsaparilla refers to several species of plants belonging to the Smilax genus, including Smilax regelii and Smilax officinalis. It has been used historically in traditional medicine for its potential health benefits, particularly for its purported detoxifying and anti-inflammatory properties.

Ingredients: Sarsaparilla contains various bioactive compounds, including saponins (such as sarsaponin and smilagenin), flavonoids, phenolic acids, and sterols. These compounds are believed to contribute to the herb's medicinal properties, including its potential as a diuretic, blood purifier, and anti-inflammatory agent.

How to Prepare: Sarsaparilla root is typically prepared and consumed as an herbal tea, decoction, or tincture. To make tea, dried sarsaparilla root is steeped in hot water for several minutes before being strained and consumed. Decoctions involve boiling the root in water to extract its active compounds, while tinctures are prepared by steeping the root in alcohol or vinegar.

Dosage: The appropriate dosage of sarsaparilla can vary depending on factors such as age, health status, and the specific preparation being used. It's important to follow the

recommended dosage on the product label or consult with a qualified herbalist or healthcare professional for personalized guidance.

How to Use: Sarsaparilla tea or tincture is typically taken orally. It's important to use sarsaparilla products as directed and to discontinue use if any adverse effects occur.

Side Effects: Sarsaparilla is generally considered safe for most people when used in moderate amounts. However, some individuals may experience allergic reactions or digestive upset. It may also interact with certain medications or have adverse effects in individuals with certain health conditions. It's important to use sarsaparilla under the guidance of a healthcare professional and to discontinue use if any adverse effects occur.

Tila:

Definition: Tila, also known as linden flower or lime blossom, refers to the flowers of the Tilia genus, primarily Tilia europaea and Tilia cordata. These trees are native to Europe, but they are also cultivated in other regions for their fragrant and medicinal flowers.

Ingredients: Tila flowers contain various bioactive compounds, including flavonoids, phenolic acids, and volatile oils. These compounds are believed to contribute to the herb's medicinal properties, including its potential as a mild sedative, anxiolytic, and anti-inflammatory agent.

How to Prepare: Tila flowers are typically prepared and consumed as an herbal tea or infusion. To make tea, dried tila flowers are steeped in hot water for several minutes before being strained and consumed.

Dosage: The appropriate dosage of tila can vary depending on factors such as age, health status, and the specific preparation being used. It's important to follow the recommended dosage on the product label or consult with a qualified herbalist or healthcare professional for personalized guidance.

How to Use: Tila tea is typically taken orally. It's often consumed in the evening as a calming bedtime beverage or during times of stress or anxiety. It's important to use tila products as directed and to discontinue use if any adverse effects occur.

Side Effects: Tila is generally considered safe for most people when used in moderate amounts. However, some individuals may experience allergic reactions or digestive upset. It may also interact with certain medications or have adverse effects in individuals with certain health conditions. It's important to use tila under the guidance of a healthcare professional and to discontinue use if any adverse effects occur.

Valerian:

Definition: Valerian, scientifically known as Valeriana officinalis, is a perennial flowering plant native to Europe and Asia. It has been used for centuries in traditional medicine for its potential calming and sedative effects.

Ingredients: Valerian root contains several bioactive compounds, including valerenic acid, valepotriates, and volatile oils. These compounds are believed to contribute to the herb's medicinal properties, including its potential as a sedative, anxiolytic, and sleep aid.

How to Prepare: Valerian root is typically prepared and consumed as an herbal tea, tincture, or capsule. To make tea, dried valerian root is steeped in hot water for several minutes before being strained and consumed. Tinctures are prepared by steeping the root in alcohol or vinegar to extract its active compounds.

Dosage: The appropriate dosage of valerian can vary depending on factors such as age, health status, and the specific preparation being used. It's important to follow the recommended dosage on the product label or consult with a qualified herbalist or healthcare professional for personalized guidance.

How to Use: Valerian tea, tincture, or capsules are typically taken orally. It's often consumed in the evening as a sleep aid or during times of stress or anxiety. It's important to use valerian products as directed and to discontinue use if any adverse effects occur.

Side Effects: Valerian is generally considered safe for most people when used in moderate amounts. However, some individuals may experience mild side effects such as drowsiness, headache, or gastrointestinal upset. It may also interact with certain medications or have adverse effects in individuals with certain health conditions. It's important to use valerian under the guidance of a healthcare professional and to discontinue use if any adverse effects occur.

Wild Cherry Bark:

Definition: Wild cherry bark, scientifically known as Prunus serotina, is the bark obtained from the black cherry tree native to North America. It has been used traditionally in Native American and folk medicine for its potential health benefits, particularly for respiratory and digestive issues.

Ingredients: Wild cherry bark contains various bioactive compounds, including cyanogenic glycosides (such as prunasin and amygdalin), flavonoids, and phenolic acids. These compounds are believed to contribute to the herb's medicinal properties, including its potential as an expectorant, cough suppressant, and mild sedative.

How to Prepare: Wild cherry bark is typically prepared and consumed as an herbal tea, decoction, or syrup. To make tea, dried wild cherry bark is steeped in hot water for several minutes before being strained and consumed. Decoctions involve boiling the bark in water to extract its active compounds, while syrups are made by simmering the bark with sugar or honey to create a thick, sweet liquid.

Dosage: The appropriate dosage of wild cherry bark can vary depending on factors such as age, health status, and the specific preparation being used. It's important to follow the recommended dosage on the product label or consult with a qualified herbalist or healthcare professional for personalized guidance.

How to Use: Wild cherry bark tea, decoction, or syrup is typically taken orally. It's often consumed to soothe coughs, sore throats, and other respiratory symptoms. It's important to use wild cherry bark products as directed and to discontinue use if any adverse effects occur.

Side Effects: Wild cherry bark is generally considered safe for most people when used in moderate amounts. However, it contains cyanogenic glycosides, which can release cyanide in the body when metabolized. While the risk of cyanide poisoning from consuming wild cherry bark is low when used appropriately, excessive intake or prolonged use may lead to adverse effects. It's important to use wild cherry bark under the guidance of a healthcare professional and to discontinue use if any adverse effects occur.

Yellowdock:

Definition: Yellowdock, scientifically known as Rumex crispus, is a perennial flowering plant native to Europe and western Asia but is also found in North America. It has a long history of use in traditional medicine, particularly among Indigenous peoples, for its potential health benefits.

Ingredients: Yellowdock root contains various bioactive compounds, including anthraquinone glycosides (such as emodin and chrysophanol), tannins, and vitamins (including vitamin A and vitamin C). These compounds are believed to contribute to the herb's medicinal properties, including its potential as a laxative, blood cleanser, and liver tonic.

How to Prepare: Yellowdock root is typically prepared and consumed as an herbal tea, tincture, or capsule. To make tea, dried yellowdock root is steeped in hot water for several minutes before being strained and consumed. Tinctures are prepared by steeping the root in alcohol or vinegar to extract its active compounds.

Dosage: The appropriate dosage of yellowdock can vary depending on factors such as age, health status, and the specific preparation being used. It's important to follow the

recommended dosage on the product label or consult with a qualified herbalist or healthcare professional for personalized guidance.

How to Use: Yellowdock tea, tincture, or capsules are typically taken orally. It's often consumed to support digestion, promote bowel regularity, and cleanse the blood. It's important to use yellowdock products as directed and to discontinue use if any adverse effects occur.

Side Effects: Yellowdock is generally considered safe for most people when used in moderate amounts. However, some individuals may experience mild side effects such as gastrointestinal upset or allergic reactions. It may also interact with certain medications or have adverse effects in individuals with certain health conditions. It's important to use yellowdock under the guidance of a healthcare professional and to discontinue use if any adverse effects occur.

Yellowdock Root:

Definition: Yellowdock root, scientifically known as Rumex crispus, is the root of a perennial flowering plant native to Europe and western Asia, also found in North America. It has a long history of use in traditional medicine, particularly among Indigenous peoples, for its potential health benefits.

Ingredients: Yellowdock root contains various bioactive compounds, including anthraquinone glycosides (such as emodin and chrysophanol), tannins, and vitamins (including vitamin A and vitamin C). These compounds are believed to contribute to the herb's medicinal properties, including its potential as a laxative, blood cleanser, and liver tonic.

How to Prepare: Yellowdock root is typically prepared and consumed as an herbal tea, tincture, or capsule. To make tea, dried yellowdock root is steeped in hot water for several minutes before being strained and consumed. Tinctures are prepared by steeping the root in alcohol or vinegar to extract its active compounds.

Dosage: The appropriate dosage of yellowdock root can vary depending on factors such as age, health status, and the specific preparation being used. It's important to follow the recommended dosage on the product label or consult with a qualified herbalist or healthcare professional for personalized guidance.

How to Use: Yellowdock root tea, tincture, or capsules are typically taken orally. It's often consumed to support digestion, promote bowel regularity, and cleanse the blood. It's important to use yellowdock root products as directed and to discontinue use if any adverse effects occur.

Side Effects: Yellowdock root is generally considered safe for most people when used in moderate amounts. However, some individuals may experience mild side effects such as gastrointestinal upset or allergic reactions. It may also interact with certain medications or have adverse effects in individuals with certain health conditions. It's important to use yellowdock root under the guidance of a healthcare professional and to discontinue use if any adverse effects occur.

Agrimony:

Definition: Agrimony, scientifically known as Agrimonia eupatoria, is a perennial herbaceous plant native to Europe, Asia, and North America. It has a long history of use in traditional medicine, particularly in European folk medicine, for its potential health benefits.

Ingredients: Agrimony contains various bioactive compounds, including tannins, flavonoids, phenolic acids, and volatile oils. These compounds are believed to contribute to the herb's medicinal properties, including its potential as an astringent, anti-inflammatory, and digestive aid.

How to Prepare: Agrimony is typically prepared and consumed as an herbal tea, tincture, or poultice. To make tea, dried agrimony leaves and flowers are steeped in hot water for several minutes before being strained and consumed. Tinctures are prepared by steeping the herb in alcohol or vinegar to extract its active compounds.

Dosage: The appropriate dosage of agrimony can vary depending on factors such as age, health status, and the specific preparation being used. It's important to follow the recommended dosage on the product label or consult with a qualified herbalist or healthcare professional for personalized guidance.

How to Use: Agrimony tea, tincture, or poultice is typically taken orally or applied topically. It's often consumed to soothe gastrointestinal issues, such as indigestion and diarrhea, or used externally to treat skin conditions.

Side Effects: Agrimony is generally considered safe for most people when used in moderate amounts. However, some individuals may experience allergic reactions or gastrointestinal upset. It may also interact with certain medications or have adverse effects in individuals with certain health conditions. It's important to use agrimony under the guidance of a healthcare professional and to discontinue use if any adverse effects occur.

Alfalfa:

Definition: Alfalfa, scientifically known as Medicago sativa, is a flowering plant in the pea family native to Asia but cultivated worldwide. It's primarily grown as fodder for livestock, but it has also been used in traditional medicine for its potential health benefits.

Ingredients: Alfalfa contains various bioactive compounds, including vitamins (such as vitamin A, vitamin C, and vitamin K), minerals (including calcium, magnesium, and potassium), amino acids, and phytoestrogens. These compounds are believed to contribute to the herb's medicinal properties, including its potential as a nutritive tonic, diuretic, and hormone balancer.

How to Prepare: Alfalfa is typically consumed as sprouts, herbal tea, or in supplement form (such as capsules or tablets). To make tea, dried alfalfa leaves are steeped in hot water for several minutes before being strained and consumed.

Dosage: The appropriate dosage of alfalfa can vary depending on factors such as age, health status, and the specific preparation being used. It's important to follow the recommended dosage on the product label or consult with a qualified herbalist or healthcare professional for personalized guidance.

How to Use: Alfalfa sprouts, tea, or supplements are typically taken orally. It's often consumed as a dietary supplement to support overall health and well-being, as well as to promote kidney health and hormone balance.

Side Effects: Alfalfa is generally considered safe for most people when consumed in moderate amounts. However, some individuals may experience allergic reactions or digestive upset. It may also interact with certain medications or have adverse effects in individuals with certain health conditions, such as autoimmune diseases or hormone-sensitive conditions. Pregnant or breastfeeding individuals should consult with a healthcare professional before using alfalfa supplements. It's important to use alfalfa under the guidance of a healthcare professional and to discontinue use if any adverse effects occur.

Ashwagandha:

Definition: Ashwagandha, scientifically known as Withaniasomnifera, is a small shrub native to India, the Middle East, and parts of Africa. It has a long history of use in Ayurvedic medicine for its potential health benefits, particularly for its adaptogenic properties.

Ingredients: Ashwagandha root contains various bioactive compounds, including alkaloids (such as withanolides), steroidal lactones, and flavonoids. These compounds are believed to contribute to the herb's medicinal properties, including its potential as an adaptogen, anti-inflammatory, and immune-modulating agent.

How to Prepare: Ashwagandha is typically consumed as a powdered root, herbal tea, tincture, or in supplement form (such as capsules or tablets). To make tea, dried ashwagandha root is steeped in hot water for several minutes before being strained and consumed.

Dosage: The appropriate dosage of ashwagandha can vary depending on factors such as age, health status, and the specific preparation being used. It's important to follow the recommended dosage on the product label or consult with a qualified herbalist or healthcare professional for personalized guidance.

How to Use: Ashwagandha powder, tea, tincture, or supplements are typically taken orally. It's often consumed to support stress management, promote relaxation, and boost overall vitality and well-being.

Side Effects: Ashwagandha is generally considered safe for most people when used in moderate amounts. However, some individuals may experience mild side effects such as gastrointestinal upset or drowsiness. It may also interact with certain medications or have adverse effects in individuals with certain health conditions, such as autoimmune diseases or thyroid disorders. Pregnant or breastfeeding individuals should consult with a healthcare professional before using ashwagandha supplements. It's important to use ashwagandha under the guidance of a healthcare professional and to discontinue use if any adverse effects occur.

Astragalus:

Definition: Astragalus, scientifically known as Astragalus membranaceus, is a flowering plant native to China and Mongolia but also found in other parts of Asia. It has been used for centuries in traditional Chinese medicine for its potential health benefits, particularly for its immune-enhancing properties.

Ingredients: Astragalus root contains various bioactive compounds, including polysaccharides, saponins (such as astragalosides), flavonoids, and amino acids. These compounds are believed to contribute to the herb's medicinal properties, including its potential as an adaptogen, immunomodulator, and anti-inflammatory agent.

How to Prepare: Astragalus is typically consumed as a powdered root, herbal tea, tincture, or in supplement form (such as capsules or tablets). To make tea, dried astragalus root slices are simmered in water for several minutes before being strained and consumed.

Dosage: The appropriate dosage of astragalus can vary depending on factors such as age, health status, and the specific preparation being used. It's important to follow the recommended dosage on the product label or consult with a qualified herbalist or healthcare professional for personalized guidance.

How to Use: Astragalus powder, tea, tincture, or supplements are typically taken orally. It's often consumed to support immune function, promote vitality, and enhance overall well-being.

Side Effects: Astragalus is generally considered safe for most people when used in moderate amounts. However, some individuals may experience mild side effects such as gastrointestinal upset or allergic reactions. It may also interact with certain medications or have adverse effects in individuals with certain health conditions, such as autoimmune diseases or diabetes. Pregnant or breastfeeding individuals should consult with a healthcare professional before using astragalus supplements. It's important to use astragalus under the guidance of a healthcare professional and to discontinue use if any adverse effects occur.

Black Cohosh:

Definition: Black cohosh, scientifically known as Actaea racemosa (formerly Cimicifuga racemosa), is a perennial herb native to North America. It has a long history of use in traditional Native American medicine and later in folk medicine for its potential health benefits, particularly for women's health.

Ingredients: Black cohosh root contains various bioactive compounds, including triterpene glycosides (such as actein and cimicifugoside), phenolic acids, and flavonoids. These compounds are believed to contribute to the herb's medicinal properties, including its potential as a hormone-balancing agent and its ability to relieve menopausal symptoms.

How to Prepare: Black cohosh is typically consumed as a powdered root, herbal tea, tincture, or in supplement form (such as capsules or tablets). To make tea, dried black cohosh root is steeped in hot water for several minutes before being strained and consumed.

Dosage: The appropriate dosage of black cohosh can vary depending on factors such as age, health status, and the specific preparation being used. It's important to follow the recommended dosage on the product label or consult with a qualified herbalist or healthcare professional for personalized guidance.

How to Use: Black cohosh powder, tea, tincture, or supplements are typically taken orally. It's often used by women to support hormonal balance, relieve menopausal symptoms such as hot flashes and night sweats, and promote overall well-being.

Side Effects: Black cohosh is generally considered safe for most people when used in moderate amounts. However, some individuals may experience mild side effects such as gastrointestinal upset or allergic reactions. It may also interact with certain medications or have adverse effects in individuals with certain health conditions, such as liver disease or hormone-sensitive conditions. Pregnant or breastfeeding individuals should consult with a healthcare professional before using black cohosh supplements. It's important to use black cohosh under the guidance of a healthcare professional and to discontinue use if any adverse effects occur.

Blessed Thistle:

Definition: Blessed thistle, scientifically known as Cnicusbenedictus, is an annual or biennial herb native to the Mediterranean region but also found in other parts of Europe, Asia, and North Africa. It has been used historically in traditional medicine for its potential health benefits, particularly for digestive and liver health.

Ingredients: Blessed thistle contains various bioactive compounds, including sesquiterpene lactones (such as cnicin), flavonoids, tannins, and essential oils. These compounds are believed to contribute to the herb's medicinal properties, including its potential as a digestive tonic, appetite stimulant, and liver tonic.

How to Prepare: Blessed thistle is typically consumed as an herbal tea, tincture, or in supplement form (such as capsules or tablets). To make tea, dried blessed thistle leaves and flowers are steeped in hot water for several minutes before being strained and consumed.

Dosage: The appropriate dosage of blessed thistle can vary depending on factors such as age, health status, and the specific preparation being used. It's important to follow the

recommended dosage on the product label or consult with a qualified herbalist or healthcare professional for personalized guidance.

How to Use: Blessed thistle tea, tincture, or supplements are typically taken orally. It's often used to support digestion, stimulate appetite, and promote liver health.

Side Effects: Blessed thistle is generally considered safe for most people when used in moderate amounts. However, some individuals may experience mild side effects such as gastrointestinal upset or allergic reactions. It may also interact with certain medications or have adverse effects in individuals with certain health conditions, such as hormone-sensitive conditions or bleeding disorders. Pregnant or breastfeeding individuals should consult with a healthcare professional before using blessed thistle supplements. It's important to use blessed thistle under the guidance of a healthcare professional and to discontinue use if any adverse effects occur.

Cat's Claw:

Definition: Cat's claw, scientifically known as Uncaria tomentosa, is a woody vine native to the Amazon rainforest and other parts of Central and South America. It has been used for centuries in traditional medicine by indigenous peoples for its potential health benefits.

Ingredients: Cat's claw contains various bioactive compounds, including alkaloids (such as oxindole alkaloids and quinovic acid glycosides), polyphenols, and other phytochemicals. These compounds are believed to contribute to the herb's medicinal properties, including its potential as an immune enhancer, anti-inflammatory, and antioxidant.

How to Prepare: Cat's claw is typically consumed as an herbal tea, tincture, or in supplement form (such as capsules or tablets). To make tea, dried cat's claw bark or leaves are steeped in hot water for several minutes before being strained and consumed.

Dosage: The appropriate dosage of cat's claw can vary depending on factors such as age, health status, and the specific preparation being used. It's important to follow the recommended dosage on the product label or consult with a qualified herbalist or healthcare professional for personalized guidance.

How to Use: Cat's claw tea, tincture, or supplements are typically taken orally. It's often used to support immune function, reduce inflammation, and promote overall well-being.

Side Effects: Cat's claw is generally considered safe for most people when used in moderate amounts. However, some individuals may experience mild side effects such as gastrointestinal upset or allergic reactions. It may also interact with certain medications or have adverse effects in individuals with certain health conditions, such as autoimmune diseases or bleeding disorders. Pregnant or breastfeeding individuals should consult with a healthcare professional before using cat's claw supplements. It's important to use cat's claw under the guidance of a healthcare professional and to discontinue use if any adverse effects occur.

Chickweed:

Definition: Chickweed, scientifically known as Stellaria media, is an annual herbaceous plant native to Europe but naturalized in many other parts of the world. It's often considered a common weed but has been used historically in traditional medicine for its potential health benefits.

Ingredients: Chickweed contains various bioactive compounds, including flavonoids, saponins, mucilage, and vitamins (such as vitamin C). These compounds are believed to contribute to the herb's medicinal properties, including its potential as a demulcent, anti-inflammatory, and mild diuretic.

How to Prepare: Chickweed is typically consumed as an herbal tea, infusion, or in fresh salads. To make tea, dried chickweed leaves and flowers are steeped in hot water for several minutes before being strained and consumed. It can also be used topically as a poultice or infused oil for skin conditions.

Dosage: The appropriate dosage of chickweed can vary depending on factors such as age, health status, and the specific preparation being used. It's important to follow the recommended dosage on the product label or consult with a qualified herbalist or healthcare professional for personalized guidance.

How to Use: Chickweed tea, infusion, or fresh leaves are typically taken orally. It's often used to soothe inflammation, support digestion, and promote overall well-being. Topically, chickweed can be applied to the skin to alleviate itching, irritation, or minor wounds.

Side Effects: Chickweed is generally considered safe for most people when consumed in moderate amounts. However, some individuals may experience allergic reactions or gastrointestinal upset. It may also interact with certain medications or have adverse effects in individuals with certain health conditions. Pregnant or breastfeeding individuals should consult with a healthcare professional before using chickweed supplements. It's important to use chickweed under the guidance of a healthcare professional and to discontinue use if any adverse effects occur.

Feverfew:

Definition: Feverfew, scientifically known as Tanacetum parthenium, is a perennial herb native to Europe but also found in other parts of the world. It has a long history of use in traditional medicine, particularly in European folk medicine, for its potential health benefits.

Ingredients: Feverfew contains various bioactive compounds, including sesquiterpene lactones (such as parthenolide), flavonoids, and volatile oils. These compounds are believed to contribute to the herb's medicinal properties, including its potential as an anti-inflammatory, analgesic, and migraine prophylactic.

How to Prepare: Feverfew is typically consumed as an herbal tea, tincture, or in supplement form (such as capsules or tablets). To make tea, dried feverfew leaves and flowers are steeped in hot water for several minutes before being strained and consumed.

Dosage: The appropriate dosage of feverfew can vary depending on factors such as age, health status, and the specific preparation being used. It's important to follow the recommended dosage on the product label or consult with a qualified herbalist or healthcare professional for personalized guidance.

How to Use: Feverfew tea, tincture, or supplements are typically taken orally. It's often used to alleviate headaches, including migraines, and to support overall well-being.

Side Effects: Feverfew is generally considered safe for most people when used in moderate amounts. However, some individuals may experience mild side effects such as gastrointestinal upset or allergic reactions. It may also interact with certain medications or have adverse effects in individuals with certain health conditions, such as bleeding disorders or pregnancy. It's important to use feverfew under the guidance of a healthcare professional and to discontinue use if any adverse effects occur.

Ginseng:

Definition: Ginseng refers to several species of perennial plants belonging to the Panax genus, including Panax ginseng (Asian ginseng) and Panax quinquefolius (American ginseng). Ginseng has been used for centuries in traditional medicine, particularly in East Asia, for its potential health benefits.

Ingredients: Ginseng root contains various bioactive compounds, including ginsenosides, polysaccharides, and peptides. These compounds are believed to contribute to the herb's medicinal properties, including its potential as an adaptogen, immune enhancer, and cognitive booster.

How to Prepare: Ginseng is typically consumed as a powdered root, herbal tea, tincture, or in supplement form (such as capsules or tablets). To make tea, dried ginseng root slices are simmered in water for several minutes before being strained and consumed.

Dosage: The appropriate dosage of ginseng can vary depending on factors such as age, health status, and the specific preparation being used. It's important to follow the recommended dosage on the product label or consult with a qualified herbalist or healthcare professional for personalized guidance.

How to Use: Ginseng powder, tea, tincture, or supplements are typically taken orally. It's often used to support energy levels, enhance cognitive function, and promote overall well-being.

Side Effects: Ginseng is generally considered safe for most people when used in moderate amounts. However, some individuals may experience mild side effects such as insomnia, gastrointestinal upset, or headaches. It may also interact with certain medications or have adverse effects in individuals with certain health conditions, such as high blood pressure or diabetes. Pregnant or breastfeeding individuals should consult with a healthcare professional before using ginseng supplements. It's important to use ginseng under the guidance of a healthcare professional and to discontinue use if any adverse effects occur.

Cleavers:

Definition: Cleavers, scientifically known as Galium aparine, is a herbaceous annual plant native to Europe, North America, Asia, and Australia. It has a long history of use in traditional medicine for its potential health benefits.

Ingredients: Cleavers contains various bioactive compounds, including iridoid glycosides, flavonoids, tannins, and mucilage. These compounds are believed to contribute to the herb's medicinal properties, including its potential as a diuretic, lymphatic tonic, and mild astringent.

How to Prepare: Cleavers is typically consumed as an herbal tea, infusion, or in fresh salads. To make tea, dried cleavers leaves and stems are steeped in hot water for several minutes before being strained and consumed. It can also be used topically as a poultice or infused oil for skin conditions.

Dosage: The appropriate dosage of cleavers can vary depending on factors such as age, health status, and the specific preparation being used. It's important to follow the recommended dosage on the product label or consult with a qualified herbalist or healthcare professional for personalized guidance.

How to Use: Cleavers tea, infusion, or fresh leaves are typically taken orally. It's often used to support lymphatic drainage, promote urinary tract health, and soothe inflammation. Topically, cleavers can be applied to the skin to alleviate itching, irritation, or minor wounds.

Side Effects: Cleavers is generally considered safe for most people when consumed in moderate amounts. However, some individuals may experience allergic reactions or gastrointestinal upset. It may also interact with certain medications or have adverse effects in individuals with certain health conditions. Pregnant or breastfeeding individuals should consult with a healthcare professional before using cleavers supplements. It's important to use cleavers under the guidance of a healthcare professional and to discontinue use if any adverse effects occur.

Eucalyptus:

Definition: Eucalyptus refers to a genus of flowering trees and shrubs, primarily native to Australia but also found in other parts of the world. Eucalyptus essential oil, extracted from the leaves of certain species, has a long history of use in traditional medicine for its potential health benefits.

Ingredients: Eucalyptus essential oil contains various bioactive compounds, including eucalyptol (cineole), terpenes, and flavonoids. These compounds are believed to contribute to the oil's medicinal properties, including its potential as an expectorant, decongestant, antiseptic, and anti-inflammatory.

How to Prepare: Eucalyptus essential oil can be used in aromatherapy, diffused in the air, or diluted and applied topically to the skin. It can also be added to steam inhalations or chest rubs to help relieve respiratory symptoms.

Dosage: The appropriate dosage of eucalyptus essential oil can vary depending on factors such as age, health status, and the specific application being used. It's important to follow the recommended dosage on the product label or consult with a qualified aromatherapist or healthcare professional for personalized guidance.

How to Use: Eucalyptus essential oil can be used aromatically, topically, or internally, depending on the intended application. It's often used to alleviate respiratory congestion, soothe sore muscles, promote relaxation, and support overall well-being.

Side Effects: Eucalyptus essential oil is generally considered safe for most people when used appropriately. However, it can be toxic if ingested in large amounts and should not be applied directly to the skin without proper dilution. Some individuals may experience allergic reactions or respiratory irritation when exposed to eucalyptus oil. It's important to use eucalyptus oil with caution, especially around children and pets. Pregnant or breastfeeding individuals should consult with a healthcare professional before using eucalyptus oil. If any adverse effects occur, discontinue use and seek medical attention.

THE END

www.ingramcontent.com/pod-product-compliance
Lightning Source LLC
Chambersburg PA
CBHW082355220526
45470CB00008B/2751